Bariatric Diet Cookbook For Seniors

Tasty and Delicious Recipes For Before And After Surgery

Wals A Smith

How to use this cookbook

Using the Bariatric diet cookbook for seniors can be a straightforward and rewarding process. Here's a guide on how to make the most of this valuable resource:

1. -Understand the Basics-
   - Begin by familiarizing yourself with the fundamental principles of the Bariatric diet. Understand the emphasis on lean proteins, whole grains, and nutrient-dense foods tailored for seniors.

2. -Read the Introduction-
   - Dive into the introduction section of the cookbook. This often provides essential information about the diet's purpose, its benefits for seniors, and general guidelines for successful adoption.

3. -Explore Meal Plans-
   - Many Bariatric diet cookbooks include sample meal plans. Explore these plans to get an idea of how to structure your daily meals. These plans often provide a balanced distribution of nutrients throughout the day.

4. -Check Serving Sizes-
   - Pay attention to serving sizes and portion control recommendations. This is crucial for seniors, ensuring that

meals align with their nutritional needs while supporting weight management goals.

5. -Adapt Recipes to Preferences-
   - The cookbook may offer a variety of recipes. Feel free to adapt them to your personal preferences and dietary requirements. Swap ingredients or modify cooking methods while keeping the nutritional principles intact.

6. -Create a Grocery List-
   - Before heading to the grocery store, create a list of ingredients needed for the chosen recipes. Having a well-organized shopping list will make your shopping experience efficient and focused.

7. -Meal Preparation-
   - Plan your meals and dedicate time for preparation. Some recipes might be suitable for batch cooking, helping you save time during the week. Consider preparing ingredients in advance for convenience.

8. -Explore Snack Options-
   - Don't forget to explore the snack recipes in the cookbook. Healthy snacks play a vital role in maintaining energy levels and preventing overindulgence in less nutritious options.

9. -Stay Hydrated-
   - While the cookbook primarily focuses on meals, hydration is crucial. Ensure you're drinking an adequate

amount of water throughout the day, and consider incorporating hydrating beverages like herbal teas.

10. -Monitor Progress-
   - Keep track of your progress. Whether it's weight management, increased energy levels, or other health goals, monitoring your journey can provide motivation and insight into the positive impacts of the Bariatric diet.

-Motivational Note-
Embarking on the Bariatric diet for seniors is not just a dietary change; it's a commitment to better health and well-being. Celebrate small victories, savor the flavors of nutritious meals, and embrace this journey as an investment in a more vibrant and active lifestyle. Remember, each step towards healthier eating is a step towards a more fulfilling and enjoyable life. You have the power to nourish your body and savor the benefits of a well-balanced and purposeful diet. Cheers to your journey to a healthier you!

WELCOME

TABLE OF CONTENTS

How to use this cookbook 3

Introduction 10

Types of Bariatric Diets for Seniors 10

-Causes of Obesity in Seniors- 10

-Symptoms of Obesity in Seniors- 11

-Preventive Measures- 11

-Bariatric Diet Cookbook for Seniors- 12

CHAPTER 1 14

What to eat and not 14

Foods to Eat on a Bariatric Diet for Seniors 14

Foods to Avoid or Limit on a Bariatric Diet for Seniors 15

Shopping ingredients 17

Benefits 20

Breakfast 24

1. Protein-Packed Smoothie Bowl 24

2. Egg and Veggie Scramble 24

3. Chia Seed Pudding 25

4. Cottage Cheese and Fruit Parfait 25

5. Spinach and Feta Omelette 26

6. Whole Grain Pancakes 26

7. Yogurt Parfait with Nuts 27

8. Almond Flour Waffles 27

9. Fruit and Nut Oatmeal 28

10. Greek Yogurt and Berry Bowl 29

Lunch 30

1. Grilled Chicken Salad 30

2. Quinoa and Vegetable Stir-Fry 30

3. Salmon and Asparagus Foil Pack 31

4. Turkey and Veggie Lettuce Wraps 31

5. Mushroom and Spinach Frittata 32

6. Cauliflower Rice Bowl with Shrimp 32

7. Black Bean and Veggie Wrap 33

8. Chicken and Vegetable Skewers 34

9. Sweet Potato and Turkey Chili 34

10. Vegetable and Chicken Sauté 35

Dinner 36

1. Baked Lemon Herb Salmon 36

2. Turkey and Vegetable Skillet 36

3. Cauliflower and Broccoli Casserole 37

4. Chicken and Vegetable Stir-Fry 37

5. Zucchini Noodles with Pesto Shrimp 38

6. Eggplant and Tomato Bake 39

7. Shredded Chicken Lettuce Wraps 39

8. Mushroom and Spinach Stuffed Chicken Breast 40

9. Tomato Basil Soup with Turkey Meatballs 41

10. Greek Salad with Grilled Chicken 41

Snacks.. 43

1. Greek Yogurt and Berry Parfait 43

2. Cucumber and Hummus Bites................................ 43

3. Cheese and Apple Slices 44

4. Roasted Chickpeas 44

5. Yogurt-Covered Frozen Grapes 45

Conclusion... 46

Introduction

A Bariatric diet for seniors is tailored to address the nutritional needs and challenges that come with age and obesity. This specialized diet aims to promote weight loss and overall health in seniors who have undergone bariatric surgery or those managing obesity through dietary modifications.

Types of Bariatric Diets for Seniors

1. -Post-Bariatric Surgery Diet-
   - Gradual progression from liquids to solid foods.
   - Emphasis on protein intake to aid in healing and muscle preservation.
   - Limited fat and sugar intake to prevent discomfort and promote weight loss.

2. -Non-Surgical Bariatric Diet-
   - Focused on portion control and nutrient-dense foods.
   - Incorporates whole grains, lean proteins, fruits, and vegetables.
   - Emphasizes mindful eating and regular physical activity.

Causes of Obesity in Seniors

1. -Metabolic Changes-
   - Reduced metabolic rate with aging.
   - Hormonal changes affecting appetite and fat storage.

2. -Lifestyle Factors-
   - Sedentary lifestyle.
   - Poor dietary habits.

3. -Medical Conditions-
   - Certain health conditions and medications contribute to weight gain.

1. -Physical Symptoms-
   - Joint pain and reduced mobility.
   - Fatigue and breathlessness.

2. -Psychological Impact-
   - Depression and low self-esteem.
   - Social isolation.

1. -Healthy Eating-
   - Follow a well-balanced bariatric diet for seniors.
   - Focus on nutrient-dense foods to meet nutritional requirements.

2. -Regular Physical Activity-
   - Engage in age-appropriate exercises.
   - Include both aerobic and strength-training activities.

3. -Behavioral Changes-

- Develop mindful eating habits.
   - Seek support from friends, family, or support groups.
4. -Medical Monitoring-
   - Regular check-ups to monitor weight, nutrition, and overall health.
   - Adjust medications if necessary under medical supervision.

5. -Psychological Support-
   - Address emotional factors contributing to overeating.
   - Consider counseling or therapy for mental health support.

6. -Hydration-
   - Ensure adequate water intake.
   - Limit sugary beverages and alcohol.

7. -Portion Control-
   - Use smaller plates to manage portion sizes.
   - Be mindful of serving sizes to avoid overeating.

Bariatric Diet Cookbook for Seniors

1. -Recipes for Nutrient Density-
   - Include recipes rich in vitamins, minerals, and protein.
   - Incorporate a variety of colorful fruits and vegetables.

2. -Protein-Packed Meals-
   - Offer recipes with lean protein sources such as poultry, fish, and plant-based options.

- Ensure a sufficient intake of protein to support muscle maintenance.

3. -Fiber-Rich Options-
   - Include recipes high in fiber to support digestion and satiety.
   - Whole grains, legumes, and vegetables can contribute to a fiber-rich diet.

4. -Hydration Tips-
   - Incorporate recipes for hydrating meals, such as soups and stews.
   - Provide ideas for infused water and herbal teas.

5. -Mindful Eating Practices-
   - Include tips on savoring flavors and enjoying meals slowly.
   - Encourage awareness of hunger and fullness cues.

A bariatric diet cookbook for seniors should focus on promoting weight loss, addressing nutritional needs, and supporting overall health through a combination of healthy eating, regular physical activity, and behavioral changes. Tailoring recipes to meet the specific requirements and challenges of seniors will contribute to successful weight management and improved well-being.

CHAPTER 1

What to eat and not

A Bariatric diet cookbook for seniors plays a crucial role in supporting weight management and overall health post-surgery or during efforts to combat obesity. Knowing the right foods to eat and those to avoid is essential for success in achieving and maintaining weight loss goals. Here's a concise guide to foods recommended for a Bariatric diet and those that should be limited or avoided.

Foods to Eat on a Bariatric Diet for Seniors

1. -Protein-Rich Foods-
   - Lean meats: Skinless poultry, fish, lean cuts of beef or pork.
   - Plant-based proteins: Tofu, legumes, lentils, and beans.
   - Eggs and dairy: Low-fat options for a protein boost.

2. -Non-Starchy Vegetables-
   - Leafy greens: Spinach, kale, and Swiss chard.
   - Cruciferous vegetables: Broccoli, cauliflower, and Brussels sprouts.
   - Colorful vegetables: Bell peppers, tomatoes, and carrots.

3. -Whole Grains-
   - Quinoa, brown rice, whole wheat, and oats.
   - High-fiber cereals and whole-grain bread.

- Incorporate these for sustained energy and fiber content.

4. -Fruits in Moderation-
   - Berries, melons, and citrus fruits are good choices.
   - Control portion sizes to manage sugar intake.

5. -Healthy Fats-
   - Avocado, nuts, and seeds.
   - Olive oil for cooking or dressing.

6. -Dairy or Dairy Alternatives-
   - Low-fat or fat-free milk, yogurt, and cheese.
   - Fortified plant-based milk alternatives like almond or soy milk.

7. -Hydrating Beverages-
   - Water should be the primary beverage.
   - Herbal teas and infused water for variety and hydration.

8. -Smaller, Frequent Meals-
   - Focus on portion control to prevent overeating.
   - Spread meals throughout the day for sustained energy.

Foods to Avoid or Limit on a Bariatric Diet for Seniors

1. -Highly Processed Foods-
   - Avoid processed snacks, candies, and sugary treats.
   - Opt for whole, nutrient-dense foods instead.

2. -High-Sugar Foods-
   - Limit intake of sugary beverages, desserts, and candies.
   - Choose natural sweeteners in moderation.
3. -Carbonated Beverages-
   - Carbonated drinks can cause discomfort and gas.
   - Opt for still water or non-carbonated options.

4. -High-Fat and Fried Foods-
   - Limit fried foods and foods high in saturated fats.
   - Choose cooking methods like baking, grilling, or steaming.

5. -Empty-Calorie Snacks-
   - Avoid empty-calorie snacks like chips and sugary cereals.
   - Opt for nutrient-dense snacks like nuts or sliced vegetables.

6. -Large Portions-
   - Overeating can lead to discomfort and hinder weight loss.
   - Focus on smaller, well-balanced meals.

7. -Caffeine and Alcohol-
   - Limit caffeinated beverages and alcoholic drinks.
   - Choose decaffeinated options and moderate alcohol consumption.

8. -Tough or Fibrous Meats-
   - Tough meats can be challenging to digest.

- Opt for tender cuts and prepare meats in a manner that makes them easier to chew.

A Bariatric diet for seniors should prioritize nutrient-dense, protein-rich, and easily digestible foods. Avoiding processed and high-sugar items, practicing portion control, and choosing healthier cooking methods are crucial components. It's important for seniors to work closely with healthcare professionals and dietitians to create a personalized plan that meets their individual needs and promotes long-term success in weight management.

Shopping ingredients

1. -Boneless, Skinless Poultry-
   - Lean protein source that is easy to digest and versatile in recipes.

2. -Fatty Fish-
   - Salmon, mackerel, or trout provide omega-3 fatty acids for heart health.

3. -Lean Cuts of Meat-
   - Choose lean options like sirloin, tenderloin, or pork loin for protein without excess fat.

4. -Tofu and Tempeh-
   - Plant-based protein alternatives for variety.

5. -Low-Fat Greek Yogurt-
   - High in protein and a good source of probiotics for digestive health.

6. -Eggs-
   - Versatile protein option with essential nutrients.

7. -Colorful Vegetables-
   - Bell peppers, spinach, kale, and broccoli for vitamins and antioxidants.

8. -Berries-
   - Blueberries, strawberries, and raspberries offer antioxidants and natural sweetness.

9. -Avocado-
   - Healthy fats and a creamy texture for salads or spreads.

10. -Nuts and Seeds-
   - Almonds, chia seeds, and flaxseeds provide healthy fats and fiber.

11. -Quinoa-
   - Whole grain with complete protein, fiber, and essential minerals.

12. -Brown Rice-
   - Fiber-rich alternative to white rice for sustained energy.

13. -Oats-
   - High-fiber option for breakfast or baking.

14. -Leafy Greens-
   - Spinach, kale, and Swiss chard for a nutrient boost.

15. -Low-Fat Cheese-
   - Calcium-rich dairy or plant-based cheese for flavor.

16. -Herbs and Spices-
   - Fresh or dried herbs, and spices for flavor without added calories.

17. -Olive Oil-
   - Healthy monounsaturated fats for cooking or dressing.

18. -Herbal Teas-
   - Caffeine-free options for hydration and variety.

19. -Low-Sodium Broth-
   - Base for soups and stews without excess salt.

20. -Fresh or Frozen Fruits-
   - Apples, pears, or frozen berries for natural sweetness and vitamins.

When creating a Bariatric diet cookbook for seniors, these ingredients can be combined to form delicious and nutritionally balanced meals. It's essential to focus on portion control, variety, and meeting individual nutritional needs. Additionally, consulting with a healthcare professional or dietitian is advisable to ensure the diet plan aligns with specific health goals and requirements.

Benefits

Following a Bariatric diet cookbook for seniors can offer numerous benefits tailored to address the specific needs and challenges associated with age and obesity. Here are some core benefits of adhering to a Bariatric diet:

1. -Weight Management-
   - Promotes gradual and sustainable weight loss, aiding in the management of obesity and related health issues.

2. -Nutrient-Dense Meals-
   - Emphasizes nutrient-dense foods, ensuring seniors receive essential vitamins and minerals for overall health.

3. -Protein Intake-
   - Prioritizes protein-rich foods to support muscle maintenance, promote healing, and prevent muscle loss.

4. -Improved Digestion-
   - Incorporates easily digestible foods, reducing the risk of digestive discomfort and complications post-bariatric surgery.

5. -Balanced Nutrition-
   - Encourages a well-balanced diet, providing a mix of carbohydrates, proteins, and healthy fats to meet nutritional needs.

6. -Enhanced Energy Levels-
   - Sustains energy levels through the consumption of complex carbohydrates and balanced meals throughout the day.

7. -Blood Sugar Control-
   - Helps regulate blood sugar levels, reducing the risk of diabetes-related complications.

8. -Heart Health-
   - Promotes heart health by including heart-friendly fats, lean proteins, and fiber-rich foods.

9. -Joint Health-
   - Supports joint health by incorporating anti-inflammatory foods and managing weight to reduce stress on joints.

10. -Cognitive Function-
   - Nutrient-dense foods contribute to brain health, potentially aiding in maintaining cognitive function in seniors.

11. -Hydration-
- Emphasizes the importance of staying hydrated, supporting overall health and preventing dehydration-related issues.

12. -Reduced Risk of Nutrient Deficiencies-
- Ensures seniors receive a variety of nutrients, reducing the risk of deficiencies that can be common in restrictive diets.

13. -Improved Mood and Mental Health-
- Balanced nutrition can positively impact mood and mental well-being, reducing the risk of depression and anxiety.

14. -Supports Healing-
- After bariatric surgery, the diet supports the healing process by providing necessary nutrients and aiding in recovery.

15. -Portion Control-
- Teaches and encourages portion control, preventing overeating and promoting healthy weight management.

16. -Digestive Regularity-
- Incorporates fiber-rich foods to support digestive regularity and prevent constipation, a common issue in seniors.

17. -Increased Mobility-
- Weight management and a nutrient-rich diet can contribute to increased mobility and overall physical well-being.

18. -Long-Term Health Benefits-
- Establishes healthy eating habits that contribute to long-term health and well-being, reducing the risk of chronic diseases.

19. -Prevention of Nutritional Complications-
- Reduces the risk of nutritional complications commonly associated with bariatric surgery or restrictive diets.

20. -Individualized Approach-
- Can be personalized to meet the specific nutritional needs and preferences of each senior, allowing for a tailored and sustainable approach.

It aims to enhance overall well-being, improve health outcomes, and support seniors in leading active and fulfilling lives.

Breakfast

1. Protein-Packed Smoothie Bowl

- -Ingredients-
  - 1/2 cup low-fat Greek yogurt
  - 1/2 cup mixed berries (strawberries, blueberries, raspberries)
  - 1 tablespoon chia seeds
  - 1/4 cup granola (low-sugar)

- -Preparation-
  - Blend yogurt and berries, pour into a bowl.
  - Top with chia seeds and granola.

- -Nutritional Value-
  - Protein: 15g, Fiber: 8g, Calories: 250
- -Cooking Time-
  - 5 minutes

2. Egg and Veggie Scramble

- -Ingredients-
  - 2 eggs
  - 1/4 cup diced bell peppers
  - 1/4 cup spinach, chopped
  - 1 tablespoon olive oil

- -Preparation-
  - Whisk eggs and cook with vegetables in olive oil.

- -Nutritional Value-
  - Protein: 14g, Fiber: 3g, Calories: 200
- -Cooking Time-
  - 10 minutes

3. Chia Seed Pudding

- -Ingredients-
  - 2 tablespoons chia seeds
  - 1/2 cup almond milk (unsweetened)
  - 1/4 teaspoon vanilla extract
  - 1/4 cup fresh berries for topping

- -Preparation-
  - Mix chia seeds, almond milk, and vanilla. Refrigerate overnight.
  - Top with fresh berries before serving.

- -Nutritional Value-
  - Protein: 8g, Fiber: 10g, Calories: 180
- -Cooking Time-
  - Overnight, plus 5 minutes

4. Cottage Cheese and Fruit Parfait

- -Ingredients-
  - 1/2 cup low-fat cottage cheese
  - 1/2 cup mixed fruit (kiwi, pineapple, and berries)
  - 1 tablespoon sliced almonds

- -Preparation-
  - Layer cottage cheese and fruits in a glass.
  - Top with sliced almonds.

- -Nutritional Value-
  - Protein: 14g, Fiber: 4g, Calories: 220
- -Cooking Time-
  - 5 minutes

5. **Spinach and Feta Omelette**

- -Ingredients-
  - 2 eggs
  - 1/4 cup fresh spinach, chopped
  - 2 tablespoons feta cheese
  - 1 teaspoon olive oil

- -Preparation-
  - Whisk eggs, cook with spinach and feta in olive oil.

- -Nutritional Value-
  - Protein: 16g, Fiber: 2g, Calories: 230
- -Cooking Time-
  - 8 minutes

6. **Whole Grain Pancakes**

- -Ingredients-
  - 1/2 cup whole wheat flour
  - 1/2 cup almond milk (unsweetened)

- 1 egg
- 1/2 teaspoon baking powder

- -Preparation-
  - Mix ingredients, cook on a griddle.

- -Nutritional Value-
  - Protein: 9g, Fiber: 4g, Calories: 180
- -Cooking Time-
  - 15 minutes

7. Yogurt Parfait with Nuts

- -Ingredients-
  - 1/2 cup low-fat vanilla yogurt
  - 1/4 cup granola (low-sugar)
  - 1 tablespoon chopped nuts (almonds or walnuts)

- -Preparation-
  - Layer yogurt, granola, and nuts in a glass.

- -Nutritional Value-
  - Protein: 12g, Fiber: 3g, Calories: 200
- -Cooking Time-
  - 5 minutes

8. Almond Flour Waffles

- -Ingredients-
  - 1/2 cup almond flour

- 2 eggs
- 1/4 cup almond milk (unsweetened)
- 1/2 teaspoon baking powder

- -Preparation-
- Mix ingredients, cook in a waffle maker.

- -Nutritional Value-
- Protein: 10g, Fiber: 3g, Calories: 220
- -Cooking Time-
- 10 minutes

9. Fruit and Nut Oatmeal

- -Ingredients-
- 1/2 cup rolled oats
- 1/2 cup almond milk (unsweetened)
- 1/4 cup mixed dried fruits and nuts (raisins, almonds, and walnuts)

- -Preparation-
- Cook oats with almond milk, top with dried fruits and nuts.

- -Nutritional Value-
- Protein: 8g, Fiber: 5g, Calories: 230
- -Cooking Time-
- 5 minutes

10. Greek Yogurt and Berry Bowl

- -Ingredients-
    - 1/2 cup low-fat Greek yogurt
    - 1/2 cup mixed berries (strawberries, blueberries, raspberries)
    - 1 tablespoon honey (optional)

- -Preparation-
    - Combine yogurt and berries, drizzle with honey if desired.

- -Nutritional Value-
    - Protein: 15g, Fiber: 5g, Calories: 200
- -Cooking Time-
    - 5 minutes

These recipes provide a variety of flavors, textures, and nutritional benefits suitable for seniors following a Bariatric diet. Adjust portions as needed and consider individual dietary restrictions.

Lunch

1. Grilled Chicken Salad

- -Ingredients-
  - 4 ounces grilled chicken breast, sliced
  - 2 cups mixed salad greens
  - 1/2 cup cherry tomatoes, halved
  - 1/4 cup cucumber, sliced

- -Preparation-
  - Combine all ingredients in a bowl.
  - Dress with olive oil and vinegar.

- -Nutritional Value-
  - Protein: 25g, Fiber: 4g, Calories: 250
- -Cooking Time-
  - 15 minutes (for grilling)

2. Quinoa and Vegetable Stir-Fry

- -Ingredients-
  - 1/2 cup quinoa, cooked
  - 1 cup mixed vegetables (broccoli, bell peppers, carrots)
  - 2 tablespoons low-sodium soy sauce
  - 1 tablespoon olive oil

- -Preparation-
  - Stir-fry vegetables in olive oil, add cooked quinoa, and soy sauce.

- -Nutritional Value-
  - Protein: 12g, Fiber: 6g, Calories: 280
- -Cooking Time-
  - 20 minutes

3. Salmon and Asparagus Foil Pack

- -Ingredients-
  - 4 ounces salmon fillet
  - 1/2 bunch asparagus, trimmed
  - 1 tablespoon lemon juice
  - 1 teaspoon olive oil

- -Preparation-
  - Place salmon and asparagus on a foil sheet, drizzle with lemon juice and olive oil, wrap and bake.

- -Nutritional Value-
  - Protein: 22g, Fiber: 3g, Calories: 300
- -Cooking Time-
  - 20 minutes

4. Turkey and Veggie Lettuce Wraps

- -Ingredients-
  - 4 ounces ground turkey, cooked
  - 1 cup lettuce leaves
  - 1/2 cup diced tomatoes
  - 1/4 cup diced bell peppers

- -Preparation-
   - Fill lettuce leaves with cooked turkey, tomatoes, and bell peppers.

   - -Nutritional Value-
   - Protein: 18g, Fiber: 4g, Calories: 220
   - -Cooking Time-
   - 15 minutes

5. Mushroom and Spinach Frittata

   - -Ingredients-
   - 2 eggs
   - 1/2 cup sliced mushrooms
   - 1 cup fresh spinach
   - 1 tablespoon olive oil

   - -Preparation-
   - Sauté mushrooms and spinach in olive oil, pour whisked eggs over, bake until set.

   - -Nutritional Value-
   - Protein: 15g, Fiber: 3g, Calories: 230
   - -Cooking Time-
   - 15 minutes

6. Cauliflower Rice Bowl with Shrimp

   - -Ingredients-
   - 1 cup cauliflower rice, cooked
   - 4 ounces shrimp, grilled

- 1/2 cup broccoli florets
    - 1 tablespoon soy sauce

  - -Preparation-
    - Stir-fry cauliflower rice, add grilled shrimp, broccoli, and soy sauce.

  - -Nutritional Value-
    - Protein: 20g, Fiber: 5g, Calories: 260
  - -Cooking Time-
    - 15 minutes

7. Black Bean and Veggie Wrap

  - -Ingredients-
    - 1/2 cup black beans, cooked
    - 1 whole-grain wrap
    - 1/4 cup diced tomatoes
    - 1/4 cup shredded lettuce

  - -Preparation-
    - Fill the wrap with black beans, tomatoes, and lettuce.

  - -Nutritional Value-
    - Protein: 12g, Fiber: 7g, Calories: 230
  - -Cooking Time-
    - 10 minutes

8. Chicken and Vegetable Skewers

- -Ingredients-
  - 4 ounces chicken breast, cubed
  - 1/2 cup cherry tomatoes
  - 1/2 zucchini, sliced
  - 1 tablespoon olive oil

- -Preparation-
  - Thread chicken and vegetables onto skewers, grill until cooked.

- -Nutritional Value-
  - Protein: 18g, Fiber: 3g, Calories: 250
- -Cooking Time-
  - 15 minutes

9. Sweet Potato and Turkey Chili

- -Ingredients-
  - 1/2 cup ground turkey, cooked
  - 1/2 cup sweet potato, diced
  - 1/2 cup black beans, canned and rinsed
  - 1/2 cup diced tomatoes

- -Preparation-
  - Combine cooked turkey, sweet potato, black beans, and tomatoes in a pot, simmer until heated through.

- -Nutritional Value-
  - Protein: 16g, Fiber: 6g, Calories: 280
- -Cooking Time-
  - 25 minutes

10. Vegetable and Chicken Sauté

- -Ingredients-
  - 4 ounces chicken breast, sliced
  - 1 cup mixed stir-fry vegetables (bell peppers, snap peas, carrots)
  - 1 tablespoon low-sodium teriyaki sauce
  - 1 tablespoon olive oil

- -Preparation-
  - Sauté chicken and vegetables in olive oil, add teriyaki sauce.

- -Nutritional Value-
  - Protein: 20g, Fiber: 5g, Calories: 260
- -Cooking Time-
  - 15 minutes

These lunch recipes for a Bariatric diet offer a variety of flavors and nutrients while prioritizing appropriate portion sizes for seniors. Adjust ingredients based on individual dietary needs and preferences.

Dinner

1. Baked Lemon Herb Salmon

- -Ingredients-
  - 4 ounces salmon fillet
  - 1 tablespoon olive oil
  - 1 tablespoon fresh lemon juice
  - 1 teaspoon dried herbs (such as dill or thyme)

- -Preparation-
- Place salmon on a baking sheet, drizzle with olive oil, lemon juice, and sprinkle with herbs. Bake until cooked.

- -Nutritional Value-
  - Protein: 25g, Fiber: 1g, Calories: 280
- -Cooking Time-
  - 15 minutes

2. Turkey and Vegetable Skillet

- -Ingredients-
  - 4 ounces ground turkey, cooked
  - 1 cup mixed vegetables (zucchini, bell peppers, cherry tomatoes)
  - 1 tablespoon olive oil
  - 1/2 teaspoon Italian seasoning

- -Preparation-
    - Sauté turkey and vegetables in olive oil, season with Italian seasoning.

  - -Nutritional Value-
    - Protein: 20g, Fiber: 4g, Calories: 250
  - -Cooking Time-
    - 20 minutes

3. Cauliflower and Broccoli Casserole

  - -Ingredients-
    - 1 cup cauliflower florets
    - 1 cup broccoli florets
    - 1/4 cup shredded cheddar cheese
    - 2 tablespoons Greek yogurt

  - -Preparation-
    - Steam cauliflower and broccoli, mix with cheese and Greek yogurt, bake until cheese is melted.

  - -Nutritional Value-
    - Protein: 15g, Fiber: 5g, Calories: 230
  - -Cooking Time-
    - 25 minutes

4. Chicken and Vegetable Stir-Fry

  - -Ingredients-
    - 4 ounces chicken breast, sliced

- 1 cup mixed stir-fry vegetables (bell peppers, broccoli, snap peas)
- 1 tablespoon low-sodium soy sauce
- 1 tablespoon olive oil

- -Preparation-
- Stir-fry chicken and vegetables in olive oil, add soy sauce.

- -Nutritional Value-
- Protein: 22g, Fiber: 4g, Calories: 260
- -Cooking Time-
- 15 minutes

5. Zucchini Noodles with Pesto Shrimp

- -Ingredients-
- 4 ounces shrimp, grilled
- 1 cup zucchini noodles
- 2 tablespoons homemade or store-bought pesto
- 1 tablespoon grated Parmesan cheese

- -Preparation-
- Toss grilled shrimp and zucchini noodles with pesto, top with Parmesan.

- -Nutritional Value-
- Protein: 18g, Fiber: 3g, Calories: 240
- -Cooking Time-

- 15 minutes

6. Eggplant and Tomato Bake

- -Ingredients-
  - 1 small eggplant, sliced
  - 1 cup cherry tomatoes, halved
  - 1 tablespoon olive oil
  - 1/2 teaspoon Italian seasoning

- -Preparation-
- Layer eggplant and tomatoes in a baking dish, drizzle with olive oil, sprinkle with Italian seasoning, bake until tender.

- -Nutritional Value-
  - Protein: 10g, Fiber: 6g, Calories: 200
- -Cooking Time-
  - 25 minutes

7. Shredded Chicken Lettuce Wraps

- -Ingredients-
  - 4 ounces cooked shredded chicken
  - 1 cup iceberg lettuce leaves
  - 1/4 cup diced bell peppers
  - 2 tablespoons low-sodium soy sauce

- -Preparation-
  - Fill lettuce leaves with shredded chicken, bell peppers, and drizzle with soy sauce.

  - -Nutritional Value-
  - Protein: 15g, Fiber: 3g, Calories: 220
- -Cooking Time-
  - 15 minutes

8. Mushroom and Spinach Stuffed Chicken Breast

- -Ingredients-
  - 4 ounces chicken breast, pounded thin
  - 1/2 cup sliced mushrooms
  - 1 cup fresh spinach
  - 1 tablespoon olive oil

- -Preparation-
  - Sauté mushrooms and spinach in olive oil, stuff chicken and bake until cooked.

- -Nutritional Value-
  - Protein: 22g, Fiber: 3g, Calories: 270
- -Cooking Time-
  - 20 minutes

9. Tomato Basil Soup with Turkey Meatballs

- -Ingredients-
  - 1 cup tomato soup (low-sodium)
  - 4 turkey meatballs (pre-cooked)
  - 1/4 cup fresh basil, chopped
  - 1 tablespoon grated Parmesan cheese

- -Preparation-
- Heat tomato soup, add meatballs, and simmer. Top with basil and Parmesan before serving.

- -Nutritional Value-
  - Protein: 18g, Fiber: 4g, Calories: 240
- -Cooking Time-
  - 15 minutes

10. Greek Salad with Grilled Chicken

- -Ingredients-
  - 4 ounces grilled chicken breast, sliced
  - 2 cups mixed salad greens
  - 1/2 cup cherry tomatoes, halved
  - 1/4 cup cucumber, sliced
  - 2 tablespoons feta cheese

- -Preparation-
  - Combine all ingredients in a bowl.
  - Dress with olive oil and red wine vinegar.

- -Nutritional Value-
    - Protein: 24g, Fiber: 3g, Calories: 290
  - -Cooking Time-
    - 15 minutes (for grilling)

These dinner recipes for a Bariatric diet offer flavorful and nutritious options for seniors. Adjust portion sizes and ingredients based on individual preferences and dietary needs.

Snacks

1. Greek Yogurt and Berry Parfait

- -Ingredients-
  - 1/2 cup low-fat Greek yogurt
  - 1/4 cup mixed berries (blueberries, strawberries)
  - 1 tablespoon chopped nuts (almonds or walnuts)

- -Preparation-
  - Layer Greek yogurt, berries, and nuts in a glass.

- -Nutritional Value-
  - Protein: 12g, Fiber: 4g, Calories: 180
- -Preparation Time-
  - 5 minutes

2. Cucumber and Hummus Bites

- -Ingredients-
  - 1 medium cucumber, sliced
  - 2 tablespoons hummus
  - 1 tablespoon cherry tomatoes, halved

- -Preparation-
  - Top cucumber slices with hummus and cherry tomatoes.

- -Nutritional Value-
  - Protein: 5g, Fiber: 3g, Calories: 100

- -Preparation Time-
  - 5 minutes

3. Cheese and Apple Slices

  - -Ingredients-
    - 1 ounce low-fat cheese (cheddar or Swiss)
    - 1 small apple, sliced
    - 1 tablespoon almond butter (optional)

  - -Preparation-
    - Pair cheese slices with apple slices, add almond butter
if desired.

  - -Nutritional Value-
    - Protein: 7g, Fiber: 4g, Calories: 150
  - -Preparation Time-
    - 5 minutes

4. Roasted Chickpeas

  - -Ingredients-
    - 1 cup canned chickpeas, drained and rinsed
    - 1 tablespoon olive oil
    - 1/2 teaspoon paprika
    - 1/2 teaspoon garlic powder

- -Preparation-
  - Toss chickpeas with olive oil, paprika, and garlic powder. Roast until crispy.
  - -Nutritional Value-
    - Protein: 6g, Fiber: 4g, Calories: 120
  - -Cooking Time-
    - 25 minutes

5. Yogurt-Covered Frozen Grapes

  - -Ingredients-
    - 1 cup grapes, washed and frozen
    - 1/2 cup low-fat vanilla yogurt

  - -Preparation-
    - Dip frozen grapes in yogurt, place on a tray, and freeze until the yogurt is set.

  - -Nutritional Value-
    - Protein: 3g, Fiber: 1g, Calories: 80
  - -Preparation Time-
    - 10 minutes (plus freezing time)

These snack recipes are designed to provide seniors following a Bariatric diet with satisfying and nutritious options. Adjust quantities based on individual dietary needs and preferences.

Conclusion

The Bariatric diet cookbook for seniors serves as a comprehensive guide, offering a diverse array of nutrient-dense recipes tailored to support weight management and overall well-being. The carefully curated recipes prioritize lean proteins, whole grains, and a variety of fruits and vegetables, ensuring that seniors receive the essential nutrients necessary for their health. The emphasis on portion control, easily digestible foods, and mindful ingredient choices makes this cookbook an invaluable resource for those seeking sustainable weight loss and improved health outcomes.

Beyond the practical recipes, the cookbook promotes a holistic approach to senior nutrition, considering the unique challenges associated with aging and obesity. By incorporating flavorful and enjoyable meals, it aims to make the dietary transition not only manageable but also a pleasurable experience.

The benefits of adopting a Bariatric diet for seniors extend beyond weight management; they encompass enhanced energy levels, improved digestion, and support for overall physical and mental well-being. The recipes are designed to prevent nutritional deficiencies, promote joint health, and contribute to heart health, aligning with the specific needs of seniors on a weight management journey.

In embracing this Bariatric diet, seniors are not just changing their eating habits; they are investing in a healthier and more fulfilling lifestyle. The cookbook encourages individuals to savor the journey towards better health, appreciating the nourishing and delicious foods that contribute to their overall well-being. As seniors embark on this culinary adventure, they are not merely adopting a diet but embracing a pathway to a more vibrant and active life. With each meal, they are nurturing their bodies, fostering resilience, and taking a meaningful step towards a healthier and happier future.

www.ingramcontent.com/pod-product-compliance
Lightning Source LLC
Chambersburg PA
CBHW070739260726
48660CB00007B/2907